Every now and then a book comes along that is truly practical. This is a book that people can use in their everyday lives. This book is free of judgement and connects with the pulse of the people.

Darlene Baxter

Karen "Raye Queen" Little understands that we live in a day and time where consuming alcohol doesn't necessarily mean not being health conscious. I am so grateful for this little pocket guide and I consult it regularly!

Dedra Arthur

The Turn up Doctor

The drinkers guide to

good health, radiant beauty

and preventing hangovers naturally!

Karen "RayeQueen" Little, HHP

Dedication

Here's to all my fellow socialites, party goers, happy hour patrons, late night creepers, and any other drinker. To every one of us who believes they have the right to be human and the right to be healthy!

Drink responsibly!

Table of Contents

INTRODUCTION

We live in a day and time where drinking has become more acceptable than ever before. Drinking at dinner parties, business lunches, and holiday celebrations or simply winding down after work is all very normal aspects of our lives. I myself enjoy chardonnay on a regular basis. As a Holistic Health Practitioner, I have a true desire to ensure my health isn't adversely affected by drinking wine daily.

So I tried various home remedies, ancient treatments and a close relationship with a higher power to get me through some tough day afters. Apparently it worked. Usually a woman of a certain age begins to look as though she has been turning

1

up too much. But nobody ever believes that I am almost in my mid 40's or that I drink damn near every day. This tells me that the methods I am using are working. I still want to look my very best without dark circles, or sagging and dry skin. I still want to feel my best without headaches, fatigue, nausea or internal damage. I strongly believe one can enjoy cocktails without looking horrible as a result. Hence, this book was born. In this small little pocket guide you will learn the science of a hangover (without all that technical stuff), natural and safe remedies for treating a hangover and how to protect your overall health from the damage drinking alcohol can cause. As a bonus, I have included a few healthy drink recipes that will help

balance the alcohol with naturally purifying agents.

This book is a must buy for anybody who enjoys

a daily glass of wine, who drinks heavily on the

weekends, who is a social drinker or anybody who

simply wants to optimize their health.

As your turn up doctor, I want to remind you to

drink responsibly. Don't over consume, don't drink

and drive and don't forget to take responsibility for

your health as well!

THE SCIENCE OF HANGOVERS

So, you turned up last night? Feeling tired? Have a headache? A bit nauseous? I am willing to bet you have a hangover my friend. We can debate all the different reasons experts suggest about the causes of a hangover but we aren't going to do that. I'm certain you have friends or family who has offered numerous remedies; some that work and some that don't. Perhaps one day, with the way that modern medicine is going, there will be a pill that instantly get rids of your hangover but that day hasn't come yet. The only full proof way to avoid a hangover is not to drink. Until then we need to find the best way to cope with the unpleasant signs and symptoms caused by consumption of alcohol to the point of intoxication.

Typically, symptoms of hangovers begin a few hours after the cessation of drinking or when different types of alcohol are consumed simultaneously. The symptoms of a hangover can last up to a couple of days, especially the older we get. The amount it takes to trigger these symptoms varies but you're generally looking at 1.5-1.75 grams of alcoholic drink per kilogram of body weight and that's basically 5-7 drinks for most people.

Most drinkers think that hangovers are caused by dehydration but it's just not that simple. In fact, I know many who drink plenty of water as they consume liquor only to still wake up with a hangover. Preventing a hangover is way more complicated than that. I don't care if you drink the entire Atlantic Ocean. Dehydration alone is not the cause of your hangover. Please don't misunderstand what I am saying. It does most definitely contribute to hangovers but so does the disruption of biological rhythms, alcohol withdrawals and just the flat out consumption of impurities.

Biologically speaking, we all have this tiny little gland call a pituitary gland that produces an anti-diuretic hormone. This hormone naturally increases blood pressure by causing your body to retain water. But by the time you've had that first shot or tequila or sipped on that most wonderful glass of

6

chardonnay, your pituitary gland pumps out less anti diuretic hormone so you lose more water. So after you have had a night to remember, you go home, go to sleep and attempt to wake up for work the next day. But once you try to lift your head up in the morning, your head aches, and your stomach is all weird and the sun is shining so brightly that you pull the blanket over your head to block out its rays.

That's because that little hormone I told you about earlier is starting to increase to make up for the decrease caused my last night's drinking. This little off and on again game your pituitary gland is playing causes the retention of fluids. That's why some of us have swollen hands and feet, puffy faces and eyes and pounding headaches as your blood pressure once again begins to go up.

As if that' not enough, your kidneys want to play games with you too. They have to work harder which in turn increases your blood pressure and heart rate and it causes sodium retention and potassium loss. So basically alcohol stops the kidneys from reabsorbing water and the excretion of urine increases. Then your body goes crazy trying to find electrolytes to regain fluids. You have an increase in blood sugars, glucose production in your liver, your pancreas pumps out more insulin, and all of this drives your kidneys and your liver crazy. They have to work overtime and that much harder to balance out the mess you created. All of this

8

disrupts your acid-alkaline (ph) balance which ultimately puts your body into fight mode causing headaches, nausea, chills, woozy feelings, sweats, fatigue...you guessed it; A HANGOVER!

The symptoms of turning up vary from one person to another with variable intensity. But to sum it up here are the major symptoms. The loss of water results in dehydration signs like dry mouth, weakness, dizziness and headaches. The retention of sodium and loss of potassium because of frequent urination cause fatigue, nausea, vomiting, weakness and muscle pain. Alcohol inhibits glucose production and uses up glucose reserves in the liver. These decreased blood sugar levels results in fatigue, weakness and mood disturbances. Alcohol consumption can create sympathetic hyperactivity which includes tremors, increased sweating, rapid heartbeats, and increased blood pressure. So contrary to popular belief, alcohol causes a lot more than just dehydration.

NATURAL HANGOVER REMEDIES

There is no 100% guaranteed way to eliminate a hangover but I have listed some tried and true methods that have proven effective in lessening the effects of turning up. Please remember that all of us are very different people with different metabolic and blood types which means that what may work for you will not work for another. I highly encourage you to try several methods until you find the one that works for you.

WATER

I will start off with hydration. You will feel miserable until you are rehydrated. Drinking enough water will ensure your proper absorption of the remaining methods. It is important to stay hydrated while you're drinking alcohol. Drink plenty of water between cocktails. If you forget, which of course is a side effect of turning up, drink plenty of water upon waking. The best water to drink is alkaline water that has a ph of 9 or above. If you don't have alkaline water you can naturally alkaline by adding 2 teaspoons of fresh lemon juice to a glass of water and sip slowly. Lemons are high in vitamin C which helps in increasing the breakdown of alcohol within the body. They also help regulate the blood sugar level. You also need to drink electrolyte rich fluids. Drinks that are high in electrolytes tend to be sports drinks, coconut water, vitamin water, and energy drinks. I don't recommend drinking energy drinks regularly but they are rich in glucose and electrolytes which relieve symptoms associated to dehydration caused by alcohol intake. Glucose provides energy and restores the blood sugar level in the body.

ACTIVATED CHARCOAL

Next on the list is my personal favorite: activated charcoal. Activated charcoal is a highly absorbent material with millions of tiny pores that capture, bind and remove poisons, heavy metals, chemicals, and intestinal gases. The porous surface has a negative electric charge that attracts positively charged unwanted toxins and gas. It is of the utmost importance to eliminate the toxins consumed when drinking alcohol. Taking activated charcoal is probably the best method I have come across for helping your hangover. Activated charcoal helps unwanted bacteria move through your system faster before they spread and multiply which helps you feel much better much faster. In fact, I have

14

taken activated charcoal to treat a hangover and ended up feeling better than I do on sober days. Just a FYI, charcoal also helps to relieve digestive issues like gas and bloating. It is most helpful if you take one charcoal tablet prior to drinking and one the morning after.

BAKING SODA

Yes Baking Soda. The same one your grandmother keeps in her refrigerator. Just make sure you are consuming pure baking soda. You will know it is pure because there will be a nutrition label on the box. Baking Soda is the go to hangover remedy if you are experiencing symptoms such as nausea and queasiness. The increased urination caused by turning up results in bicarbonate loss. Guess what Baking Soda is? You guessed it; sodium bicarbonate. This makes it the ideal natural cure for hangovers. Alcohol increases the acidity of the stomach. Baking soda neutralizes the acid and reduces the stomach symptoms of hangovers. Mix ½ teaspoon of baking soda in a glass of water to reduce the acidity in your body. You can do these several times throughout the day until symptoms subside. Take this mixture on an empty stomach 15 minutes before eating.

CAYENNE PEPPER AND OTHER SPICES

There are certain foods and spices that encourage detoxification by breaking down alcohol and stimulating liver function. Look to spicy foods to heat things up and sweat them out. By consuming spicy food you help your body release get rid of pesky hangover-causing toxins. Secondly, spicy foods will make you drink more water. The more water you drink the quicker you can rehydrate.

HANGOVER FIGHTING FOODS

Before Going Out

Let's talk before and after. Before going out for a night on the town eats foods that contain high amounts of fatty acids such as

1. avocados

2. salmon

3. hemp oil

4. walnuts

5. almonds

6. dark green leafy vegetables

7. olive oil

8. flaxseed oil

9. whole grain foods

10. lean meats

11. eggs

One longstanding folk remedy is to take a spoonful of olive oil before drinking. The grease in these fatty acids are said to coat the intestines so the alcohol takes longer to absorb giving you more time to flush the toxins out of your system.

FOODS THE MORNING AFTER

But if you didn't get a chance to enjoy your salmon dinner before going out there is still hope. There are certain foods that have natural hangover fighting chemicals that will help ease the symptoms the morning after.

1. Ginger has been used for centuries by people globally. It is one of the most popular natural cures for nausea and vomiting and digestive distress caused by excessive intake of alcohol. Ginger soothes the digestive tract and balances the gastric juices. Try nibbling crystallized ginger in the aftermath of a night

of drinking or drink of ginger ale or ginger tea.

2. Apples are a great choice for a hangover because they are high in fructose, a fruit sugar that helps metabolize alcohol quickly and have headache-fighting qualities.

3. Vegetables like asparagus are rich in amino acids and minerals that speed up the metabolism of alcohol and help protect your cells.

4. Because you become vitamin-deficient while drinking, tomatoes are great to eat when you're hung over because they're hydrating, high in vitamin C and B and water.

5. Surprisingly, chicken noodle soup isn't just for the common cold. Chicken noodle soup is a great hangover food because it is hydrating and it restores sodium levels. The vegetables in soup contain phytonutrients and other micronutrients that help fight inflammation which is a common side effect when drinking. Chicken contains cysteine which not only fights headaches but it supports the liver. Menudo is a popular hangover soup as well because of the spices it contains.

6. Bananas are one of the most popular go to foods for hangovers. Bananas are the obvious choice because it puts potassium into your system fast, they are gentle on the

stomach and they provide electrolytes lost during turning up.

7. Cabbage – Not only can cabbage heal stomach ulcers but it also absorbs alcohols acetaldehyde and is known to relieve headaches due to lactic acid. Cabbage is thought to clear the body of congeners. Congeners are the toxic by-products of the fermentation process. You can simply eat cabbage or you can try the method our ancestors swear by; boil some cabbage and save the juice to drink the morning after a night out.

VITAMINS

Ok. Aside from the fact that most of us should be taking vitamins on a daily basis anyway, you should most certainly be taking them to recover from a hangover. Remember when we discussed that alcohol is a diuretic which means you not only loose water but you also loose vitamins and nutrients while you are partying. Let's start with the most important one; B and C Vitamins. B1, better known as thiamine, help prevent the buildup of a chemical in the brain which may be associated with headache you experience during your hangover. B12 performs a key role in the functioning of the brain and nervous system and will help combat fatigue. And by simply replacing the B2, and B6, you will simply feel better. Consider taking a B complex vitamin both before and after a night out on the town. Regular drinkers swear by B Vitamins. Vitamin C helps you to detox by fighting free radicals your body is loaded with as a result of drinking. It wouldn't hurt to add a Vitamin A supplement as well, I'm just saying.

REFLEXOLOGY

These are the simplest reflexology hangover relief tricks ever. It ACTUALLY works. You can rub your hangover away. Please don't knock it until you try it.

Reflexology Trick #1

This is always performed on the second toe on each food. In case you are too hung over to remember, the second toe is next to the big toe. Now, just under the toe nail, opposite side of the big toe, is a small pressure point area that leads to the energy pathway that travels straight through your stomach. This energy pathway is blocked and sluggish because of dehydration. All you have to do is get the energy to flow again so the blockages from drinking too much are removed. So simply use on finger to gently but firmly push down in a circular motion for about two minutes one way and then two minutes the other way. Always do the right foot first and then do the left. Repeat as much as needed until you begin to feel relief.

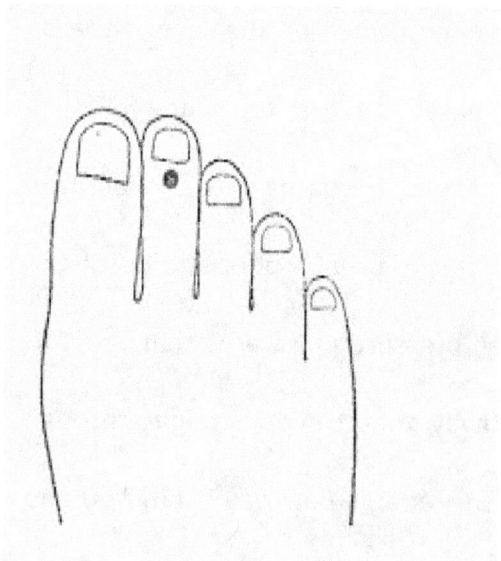

Reflexology Trick #2

Stimulate the outer edge area on the right foot followed by kneading the middle of your foot and pressing your little toe.

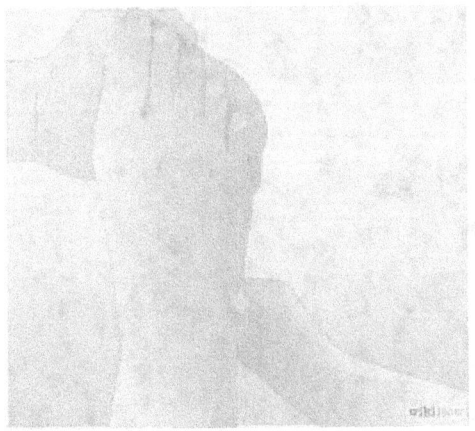

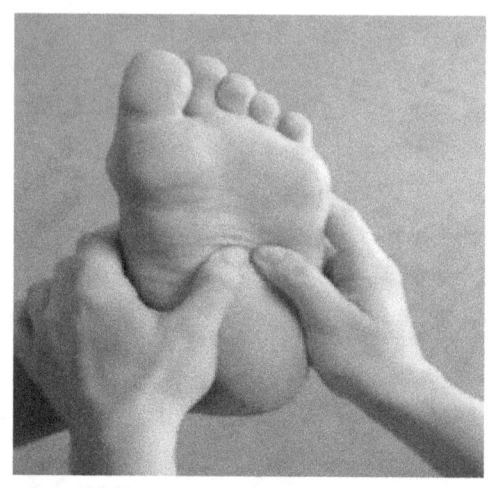

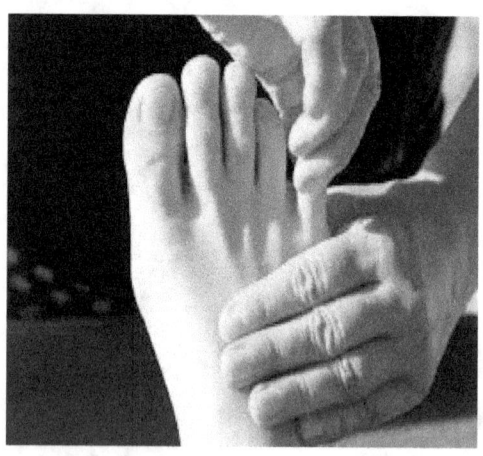

Reflexology Trick #3

Run your wrists under water. This trick works exceptionally well if you are suddenly feeling sick. Depending on how much alcohol is consumed, you can use this trick for up to 3 minutes at a time to start to feel better. Not only will this trick help to subside nausea but it will also take away sweating and begin to cool the body from the inside out. Simply place your wrists under cool or cold water for 30 seconds to 3 minutes.

Reflexology Trick #4

Ok ok ok. I get it. The morning after isn't the best time to try to bend over and reach your feet. If you are finding it too difficult to reach your feet without feeling dizzy then perhaps you should opt for hand reflexology. There are some pressure points in the hand that will help to ease your hang over symptoms as well. The first one will help reduce nausea. Simply apply pressure on your left wrist using your thumb. Rotate for about 3 minutes each way. Then place your index finger and middle finger on the back of your wrist. Apply pressure and rotate for about 3 minutes each way.

FOR NAUSEA

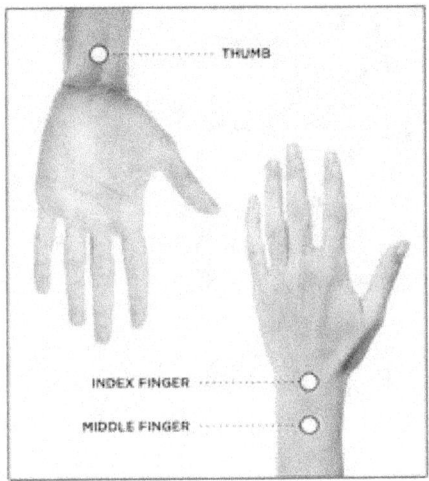

Reflexology Trick #5

The final reflexology trick I want to share with you is also one that is performed on the hand. Squeeze the tips of your index finger and your thumb finger together. You will see a little muscle bulge when you do this. Simply apply pressure.

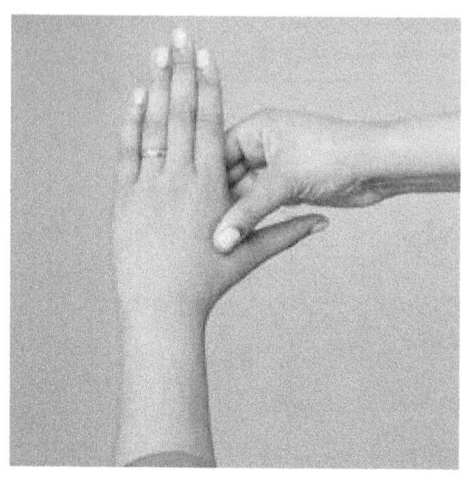

Please be mindful that although reflexology is safe for most people, there are a few select people who shouldn't try it. If you are suffering from deep vein thrombosis, cellulite on the feet or legs, have had a stroke in the last 2 weeks, an acute infection with high temperature, an unstable pregnancy or pregnancy within the first trimester, epilepsy, insulin dependent diabetics, lymphoma patients, people taking anti-coagulating drugs, or people with

contagious conditions. And remember that water is

extremely important to reflexology and it is vital to

have a large glass of water every time you practice

reflexology.

BEAUTY AND THE DRINK

It's no secret that alcohol accelerates the aging process. We look amazingly beautiful when we hit the town but trust me; you will begin to look like you should be turning down instead of turning up unless you take some precautions. Alcohol worsens the skin, causes bloating, affects our eyesight, and damages your hair. But never fear I have precautions that are simple, inexpensive and necessary. So let's do it.

THE EYES HANG OVER

Alcohol causes broken capillaries in your eyes. It irritates and enlarges the tiny blood vessels on the surface of your eye causing a "bloodshot" appearance. Excessive drinking even robs the body of some nutrients require to maintain eye health and could possibly lead to blindness. I think the most obvious eye hang over is the oh-so-beautiful dark circles under eyes and eye puffiness. This is the look that nobody wants. So how do we get rid of the eye hang over? There are some basic things that should be done like getting plenty of sleep and drinking extra water.

Cucumbers

In addition to that there are some age old tricks that are tried and true like placing cucumber slices over each eye while lying down which can refresh the skin and reduce puffiness. Cucumbers immediately hydrate the eyes and reduce eye swelling. Cucumbers also happen to be rich in nutrients that helps nourish the skin around the eyes and gets rid of dark under eye circles. The Vitamin C and the coolness from the cucumber constrict blood vessels which reduce the swelling and relieve the redness. Leave the slices over the eyes for about 10 minutes. You can substitute cucumbers with tea bags or ice cubes wrapped in a soft cloth. The tannin in tea bags will help reduce swelling and well as discoloration.

Aloe Vera Gel and Vitamin E

Aloe Vera has many anti-inflammatory and healing properties. Use aloe vera gel mixed with vitamin E oil and apply it on the swollen area. This can be left on overnight for best results. Aloe and vitamin E will also treat infections on the skin and eyes and reduces the appearance of wrinkles.

Almond Oil

Gently massage almond oil on the affected areas of your eye. For best results do this at night and leave on overnight.

Rose Water

Soak cotton pads in rose water and keep them over your eyes for about 5 minutes. Rose water is one of the best remedies to remove dark circles under eyes as it lightens the skin and acts as a natural soothing agent.

THE SKIN HANG OVER

Drinking alcohol is one of the main culprits of rosacea, psoriasis, dryness, wrinkles, saggy skin and acne. Bet you didn't know that. Alcohol not only increases blood flow and dilates the tiny blood vessels that are closest to the outer layer of your skin but sometimes they burst. Skin that is dry from the inside wrinkles faster, turns pale or ashy, and robs the skin of Vitamin A- an antioxidant that is necessary for cell renewal and turnover. The dehydrating effect of alcohol and depletion of all anti-oxidants makes the skin susceptible to free radical-induced damage which results in hyperpigmentation, coarse texture, wrinkles and more. The bottom line is you will age faster if you aren't mindful.

Dull and Dry Skin

Turning up too often can lead to your skin looking dull, gray, and acne prone. Another contributor to the over-time ugly skin is falling asleep with make-up on. Dull skin can make your skin look tired and old. There are a few DON'TS you can do to prevent dull skin. First off, do NOT fall asleep with make-up on. This causes a lot of stress on facial skin which leads to breakouts and dull skin. Make certain you thoroughly wash your face after a night out on the town. Do not eat junk food at 4 in the morning because alcohol is processed first which means the junk food stays in your system longer causing skin eruptions. So you got really drunk last night and you forgot to take your make up off (or maybe you didn't go straight to sleep) hmmmm. We can't worry about last night. Let's focus on now. So how can you revive your dull skin? First, always eat fresh fruits and vegetables. Eat a few servings a day to naturally revive your dull skin.

Honey and Sugar Exfoliation

The first step to getting rid of your lifeless skin is to remove all dead skin cells by exfoliating. An easy recipe to do this is to mix some honey and sugar granules in a bowl. Rub it on your face and neck. Rub gently to remove dead skin and then wash your face with water. Do this once a week to give your skin that natural glow.

The Lemon Mask

My personal favorite is the lemon mask. The lemon mask will give a natural glow to your skin. All you have to do is squeeze the juice out of a lemon and apply it on your face or you can simply cut a lemon in half and squeeze it while rubbing it all over your face. Be very careful to avoid the eye area. Let this sit for 15 minutes. If you find the lemon mask to be over drying add some olive oil, almond oil or honey to your face as well.

The Almond Mask

How easy is this? Simply rub a generous amount of almond oil all over your face. Let it sit for about 15 minutes with a steamy rag on top of your face. Wash and go. Voila!

Wrinkles and Saggy Skin

Excessive alcohol leads to dehydration which leads to a host of other problems including wrinkles...yes wrinkles not to mention fine lines. Come on now, you don't want people to think you and your mother are sisters (unless she looks really really young). Heavy drinking can lead to saggy facial features and the loss of skin elasticity. The first thing you must do to avoid wrinkles is to drink water. I know I have said this a million times already but it's the truth. Water is the basis for everything our bodies need. Then consider this perfect age old mask.

Egg White Mask

Egg whites are a natural astringent. It contains hydro lipids which help lift loose skin. It's super easy to make. All you have to do, even if you are hung over, is whisk one to two egg whites until you get a foamy texture. Apply it to the face and neck. Leave it on for about 20 minutes and then rinse with cool water. Use this twice a week to enjoy firm, radiant skin. You can also use lemon or honey in the place of egg white to achieve similar results.

The Mother Mask

Vitamin C is the mother of mothers. It helps produce collagen in the skin. Collagen is what keeps our skin young and wrinkle free. After about the age of 20 we start to loose collagen so it becomes necessary to replace it. Vitamin C will help fade age and sun spots and it has the muscle to fight off all those free radicals that cause us to age prematurely. Vitamin C is the truth! All you have to do is mix a pure form of vitamin c which should read as L. Ascorbic Acid. Thinks of love that way you won't forget the L in front of Ascorbic. No L no go! Simply mix your pure form of Vitamin C with glycerin, distilled water, coconut oil, jojoba oil or Vitamin E oil. Leave it on for about 5-10 minutes to have radiant, lighter, brighter, tighter and softer skin.

The Healthy Hangover

Now let's discuss taking care of the ugly on the inside. Our organs are the keys to longevity and a good quality of life. If you enjoy turning up then you should pay particular attention to the health of your liver and kidneys. This chapter will provide you with some simple and natural remedies to ensure you protect your health from the inside out. I have experimented with a lot of different healthy hangover remedies in an attempt to preserve my health. I will share with you the ones I have found to be the most beneficial and effective as reported by myself, my clients and popular research.

Let's start with the need to feed your body potassium. As mentioned earlier, your body rids itself of potassium when drinking so it is only logical to replenish the potassium lost. Most of us know when we are going to be drinking so if you overload your body with lots of potassium leading up to your night out your body will thank you. Coconut water is indeed one of the best methods for quickly getting potassium into your body followed by eating bananas. You should do this both before and after drinking for your body to enjoy the nutritional benefits. You can also visit your local health food store and purchase effervescent electrolyte tablets.

While you are at the health food store consider picking up some amino acids such as cysteine. Your body creates acetaldehyde from alcohol metabolism while you are consuming alcohol. Amino acids will help your liver break down the acetaldehyde. This will prevent your liver from working twice as hard causing unnecessary stress. You can also find cysteine from foods such as poultry, oats, dairy, red pepper, garlic, onions and wheat germ.

There are several other herbal formulas that regenerate the liver and detoxify the blood. Milk thistle, goji berry and ginger are powerful liver detox herbs. Spirulina consist of 60% of protein adding amino acid 18 types, Vitamin B and E, and Minerals to nourish the liver and to help detox.

As for the Kidneys, let's hear it for cranberries. Cranberries may be helpful for cleansing the kidneys of the excess calcium that contributes to the formation of kidney stones which is a common side effect of alcohol abuse. Now I know you are sick of hearing about the great and powerful lemon but it is such an amazing fruit. Lemon juice has been shown to increase citrate levels in the urine which helps prevent kidney stones from forming. Simply squeeze lemons into hold or cold water daily. In addition to the above remedies you should consider doing kidneys cleanse once a week. Simply add lemons, apple cider vinegar (organic and raw) and purified water and drink 3-4 times a week.

HEALTHY DRINK RECIPES

The Green Bee

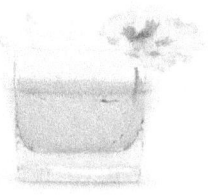

2 oz. Blue Ice Organic Wheat Vodka

1 oz. Agave Nectar

1 oz. Lemon Juice

5 mint leaves

Garnish: Lemon Zest

Tear mint into shaker. Add ice, agave nectar, lemon juice and shake vigorously. Strain into cocktail glass and garnish with lemon zest. Enjoy!

Real Green Apple Martini

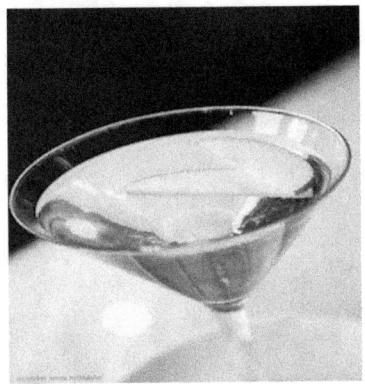

Vodka (organic is best)

Fresh organic green apples

Fresh Lime

Forget the gross corn syrup green apple mix. Simply shake organic vodka over plenty of ice and float with a slice of fresh organic green apple. Garnish with lime.

The Last Straw

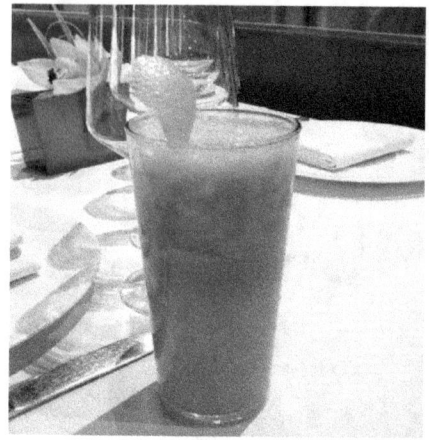

2 oz. vodka (organic is best)

Strawberries

Lemonade

Soda

Muddle strawberries in a mixing glass. Add vodka and a splash of soda and top with lemonade.

Bitter Tea

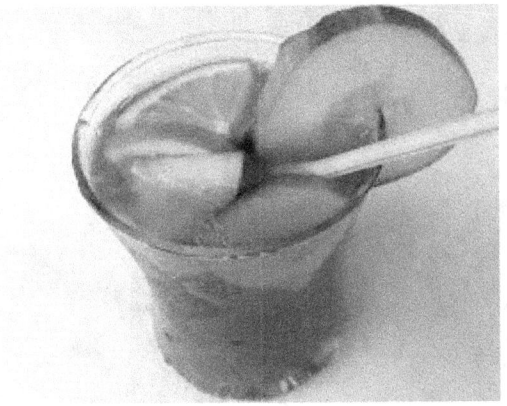

Fruity tea of your choice

½ ounce bitters

3 ounces pomegranate juice

Limes

Cucumbers

Brew a cup of fruity black tea and stir in ½ shot bitters and 1 ½ shots pomegranate juice. Add squeezed lime slices and garnish with cucumbers.

Caramel Mint Hot Chocolate

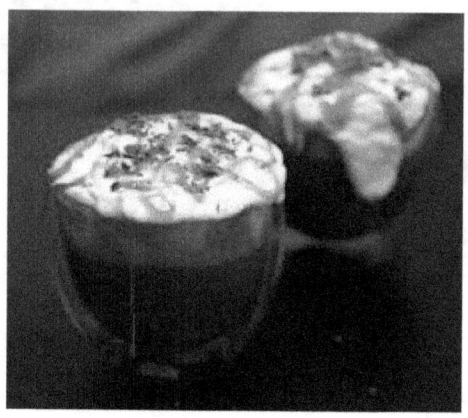

1 cup milk (Almond, soy or coconut are best)

1 packet cocoa mix

1 shot of tequila

½ shot of peppermint schnapps

Whipped cream

Organic caramel

Heat 1 cup milk and stir in 1 packet light hot cocoa mix. Add 1 shot tequila and 1/2 shot peppermint schnapps. Top with whipped cream and caramel.

Minnesota Mojito

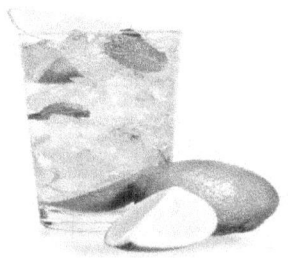

1 splash peppermint schnapps

1 oz. vodka (organic is best)

1 tbsp. honey

½ lime cut into wedges

¼ c. mint leaves

Sparkling water

Mint sprig

Muddle mint leaves, honey, lime wedges and peppermint schnapps in mixing glass. Pour mixture into glass. Add ice and vodka and top with sparkling water. Stir well and garnish with mint sprig.

White Sangria

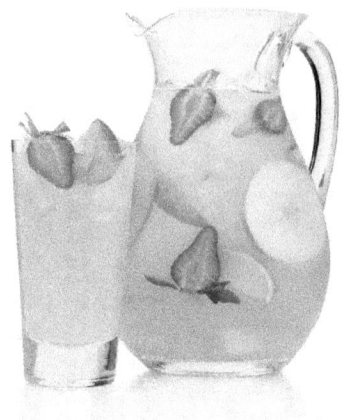

2 strawberries

½ peach

½ a pear

2 shots of white wine

¼ cup seltzer

In a wine glass, combine two strawberries (halved),
½ a fresh peach (diced), ½ a pear (diced), 2 shots
white wine, and ¼ cup seltzer.

Watermelon Martini

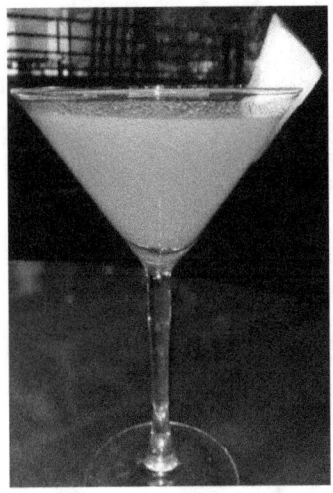

1 ½ oz. cucumber vodka

3 oz. watermelon juice

½ oz. lime juice

Watermelon slice

Combine all ingredients in a shaker filed with ice.
Shake vigorously. Strain into a martini glass and
garnish with a lime slice.

Peppermint Patty

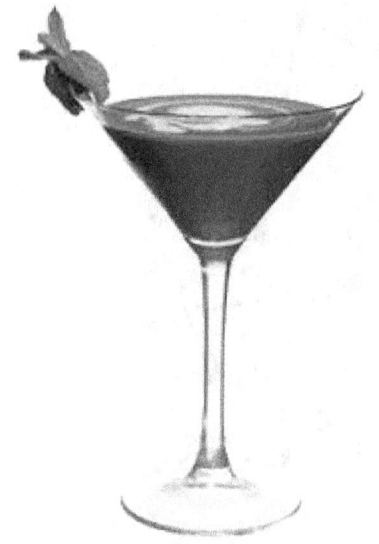

Fresh mint leaves

½ shot vodka

1 tsp. light chocolate syrup

Muddle 6 fresh mint leaves with ½ shot vodka. Add
a splash of water and 1 teaspoon light chocolate
syrup. Mix in a shaker with ice. Strain before
serving.

Caprese Martini

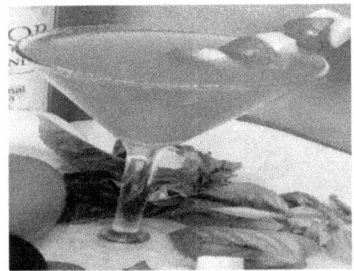

4 cherry tomato halves

2 basil sprigs

1 splash of balsamic vinegar

1 tsp. sugar

2.5 oz. tomato vodka

Garnish: cherry tomato halves and mozzarella cubes

Muddle tomatoes, basil and sugar in a mixing glass. Add vodka, vinegar and shake vigorously. Pour into a chilled martini glass and garnish with a skewer of cherry tomato halves and mozzarella cubes.

Lemon Drop

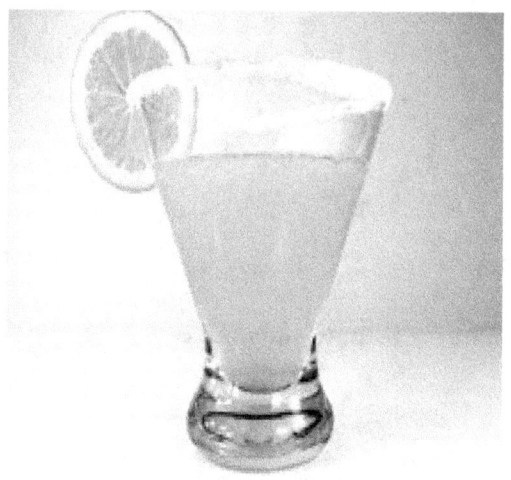

½ shot of vodka (organic is best)

½ shot fresh-squeezed lemon juice

½ tsp. honey

In a shaker with ice, combine 1/2 shot vodka, 1/2 shot fresh-squeezed lemon juice, and 1/2 teaspoon honey.

Tall Grass Tea

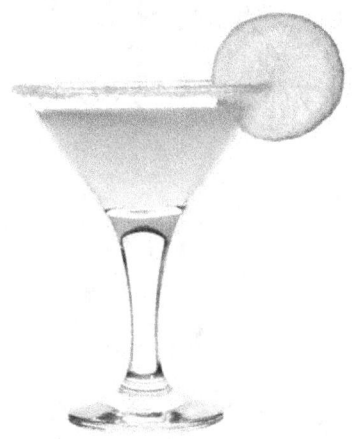

3 oz. vodka (organic is best)

4 oz. green tea

1 tbsp. sugar

2 tbsp. lemon juice

Combine ingredients in a shaker filled with ice, shake vigorously and strain into a sugar-rimmed martini glass.

Vodka Soda

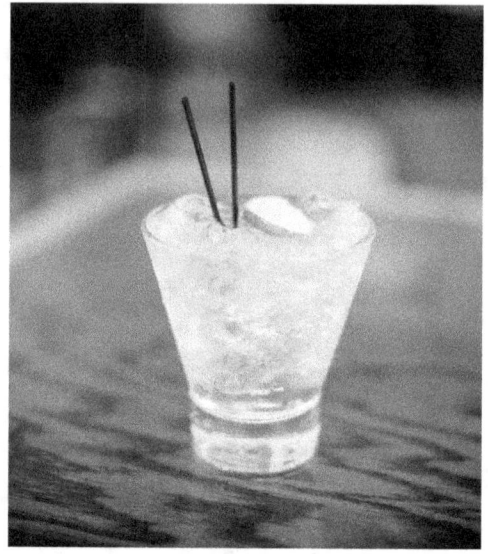

1 shot of vodka

2 shots of seltzer

Lemon or lime or both

Mix all ingredients poured ice. Garnish with a lemon
or a lime.

Rosemary Cucumber Lemonade

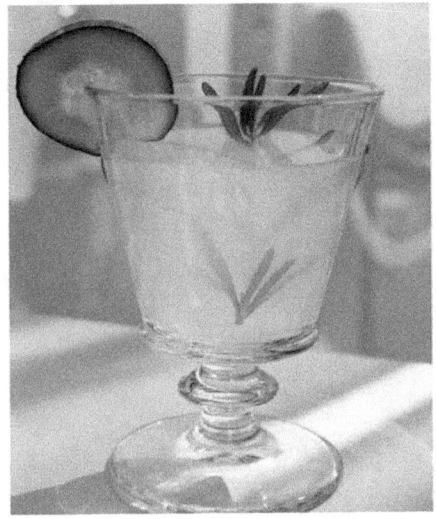

3 lemons

1 tsp. honey

1 shot vodka (organic is best)

¾ cup seltzer

Garnish: cucumber slice and rosemary sprig

Stir together juice from 3 lemons and 1 teaspoon honey. Add 1 shot vodka and ¾ cup seltzer. Garnish with a cucumber slice and a rosemary sprig.

Cape Codder

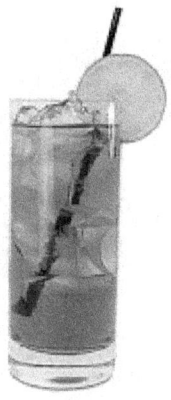

1 shot of vodka

2 shots of cranberry juice

Seltzer water

Lime

Pour 1 shot of vodka and 2 shots cranberry juice (100 percent juice, no sugar added) over ice. Add 2 shots seltzer water, stir, and garnish with a lime wedge.

CONCLUSION

I had so much fun writing this book, however, I do not want to send the wrong message. Alcoholism is a very real disease and we need to pay particular attention to how much alcohol we consume.

Contrary to popular belief beer and wine are the most toxic of adult beverages. From that point it is best to drink clear liquor as it is less toxic than its dark counterparts.

If you are someone you know has a suspected alcohol abuse problem please seek professional help.

ABOUT THE AUTHOR

Karen "RayeQueen" Little is board certified Holistic Health Practitioner, Master Nutritionist, and Holistic Therapist. Karen received her BA degree from Langston University, sought her MA in Sociology from University of Nevada at Las Vegas and her post graduate certification from Natural Healing College. Karen "RayeQueen" is the proud mother of 2 wonderful boys, K'Saan Thompson and Austin Kelly. As a former school teacher and devout community member, Karen has a true passion for the health and well-being of her people and all people. Karen "RayeQueen" has also written *The Secret for Sistahs* and *The Majortarian.*

Karen "RayeQueen" Little currently operates her

private practice out of Denver, Colorado and is the

chief practitioner of Peace of Mind Spiritual Center.